42 Weight Loss Tips
Your Life

C000135892

by Andreas M

42 Weight Loss Tips That Will Change Your Life Forever.

ISBN: 978-9963-277-04-9
Cyprus Library.
www.cypruslibrary.gov.cy

Table of Contents

About the Author 1

Prologue 2

Start walking 5

Walking and Running 7

Running baby, yes! Oh yes! 9

Eat lots of small meals during the day. 11

Drink water the moment you wake up. 12

Finish eating at least 2 hours before bed time..........................15

Drink water 30 minutes before having a meal. 16

Never eat fruit after a meal containing carbs or meat. 17

Apply mono-food eating. 18

Water fast at least once a week. 19

Colon cleansing at least every two months. 20

Replace white sugar with brown sugar. 21

Replace white flour with whole wheat flour..............................23

Replace White Salt with Pink Salt or Low Sodium Salt.................23

Replace animal milk with plant based milk 24

Replace white rice with brown rice. 26

Eliminate oils from your diet. 27

Replace Processed Carbs with natural ones. 28

Gradually reduce your meat consumption. 29

Gradually reduce sodas and sugary drinks from your diet. 31

Gradually reduce and eliminate coffee from your diet. 32

Breathing exercises. 35

Stop watching TV. 36

Stop Wasting your time with Social Media. 36

Start watching Nutritionfacts. org videos. 37

Buy these Books. 38

Download these free books. 39

Start learning from these doctors and dieticians. 39

Stop going to junk food restaurants. 40

Increase your fruit consumption. 42

Increase your vegetable consumption......................................43

Increase your legume consumption. 44

Increase your Starch consumption. 45

Increase your nuts consumption...47
Drink more smoothies. 48
Get 8 hours of sleep. 48
Keep a Food Diary..50
Keep an Exercise Diary. 51
Set Goals and work "Religiously" to accomplish them.................52
Never stop searching and questioning. 53
Be a little selfish..55
A journey starts with a small step. 56
Other books by Andreas Michaelides. 59

Find more about me and my books at my webpage www.thirsty4health.com

About the Author

Andreas was born in Athens, the city that gave birth to Democracy, in Greece, the country that taught to the world how to live, think, and have fun. He grew up in the beautiful island of Cyprus.

With both of his parents bibliophiles (and his father a high school teacher), Andreas grew up with a love and appreciation for literature. In addition to the books he borrowed from the school library, a stack of encyclopedias taught him about the world. A history lover from age 13, he devoured the memoirs of Winston Churchill and Charles de Gaul, and by age 17, he had read all of Julius Vern's books.

After serving his country for 26 months immediately after finishing high school, Andreas studied in Patra, Greece to become a computer engineer. With his Master of Computer Engineering and Informatics, he began working in the Informatics Department of the local university hospital, and started reading again with a vengeance.

In 2004, Andreas authored his first book, a historical novel that has not yet seen the light of publication. Leaving it unpublished made him feel like a failure, but a lot has changed since then. Eleven years later, he has successfully quit smoking and has been smoke-free for the past six years. He has also started running again and managed to lose 26 kg (57 lbs).

Andreas has run three marathons, as well as many half-marathons and other shorter races. His love for running is what renewed him and actually saved his life.

Multiple medical problems pushed Andreas to research and experiment with a plant-based diet; since 2013 he is following a whole plant based diet.

In addition to running, Andreas enjoys hiking, cycling, playing basketball, camping, photography, and going out with friends and family and having a good time.

Prologue

This story is going to be long, so if you don't like lengthily reading, then maybe, you'll keep struggling with weight loss. However, if you don't want such thing to continue, keep reading till the end.

One of the first things I did when I was overweight and decided I had enough was to order from Amazon a lot of books about weight loss, many of them were hocus pocus, others were ok, and some of them were amazing.

That's why in my books, I try to deliver information that the reader, that's you, will find useful and also be able to apply it immediately or at a reasonable pace.

I am a very practical man; I will read the theory as long as I can see the usefulness of it and also the practical applications that it offers.

I am more of a hands-on person than a day-dreamer, which was what I was when I was overweight and had some chronic diseases, which made my life miserable and reduced its quality.

So, yes, this story is going to be long; there is no other way to pass around all the information I know, which was accumulated from books written by doctors, medical researchers, dieticians and also credible medical sites with articles reviewed and written by medical personnel. Finally, there will be information that I have acquired from my experience, from my everyday trial-and-error applications and experimentations with different kind of foods, diets, and lifestyles.

Back in 2010, I decided that I was not going to be a fat, sick man anymore, and I took my life into my own hands.

The amazing thing is not just losing the pounds -after all, so many people out there reading these lines are shaking their heads because they have done it so, lost the pounds - but it's the lack of knowledge of how to avoid getting them back.

Well, my amazing people, I have that knowledge, not only did I lose 44 pounds, but I never gained them back. Most importantly, I lost the pounds in a healthy way, and I never starved myself to do it. How I did it is briefly described in one of my latest very short books, which you can read in under one hour: *My Weight Loss Journey: How I lost 44 pounds and never gained them back, using a plant-based diet.*

In these lines, you are going to discover 42 weight loss tips that if you follow them, you will see long-term results.

I do not believe in miracles; miracles are for the ignorant people out there who lack the will to search and research, apply, take the risk of failure, and learn from their mistakes.

The shape of your body is a direct result of the way you think. The information you have and the willingness to acquire new data will enable you or not to first change your way of thinking and then start working on your body.

Writing this story makes me pause a lot and reminisce about how I started this beautiful journey of mine as a heavy smoker and overweight- I would smoke at least 40 cigs a day, I am 5. 9" tall, and my weight back then was 185 pounds! I was already 22 pounds overweight, and I was a chain smoker; yes I know, I was really "smart" back then. After quitting smoking, I gained another 22 pounds in a year, and I was at the magic number of 207 pounds!

The doctor that gave me my first blood test results, after I had been ignoring it for many years, told me flat on my face, and I thank him for his honesty, that it's a beautiful thing that I managed to stop smoking, but I really needed to do something about my weight. He said that I had increased chances for diabetes 2, heart condition, high blood pressure, high cholesterol, colon cancer, and a lot of other chronic diseases.

Yes, you guessed it, I ignored the doctor when he told me those things and went on with my life.

Well, I will say something that pretty much gives me an excellent excuse; I just managed to get rid of a deadly addiction, namely smoking, and I was pretty happy with my accomplishment. If you stop and think that only 7% of the people that try to quit succeed in remaining ex-smokers for the rest of their life, that was an amazing feat I had just done. For your information, I am in my seven years now smoke-free and still proud of it.

So yes, except for the tips on how to lose weight, I also know how to quit smoking and never take another puff in your life again. I briefly describe my smoking escapades in my latest book, *16 Common Smoking Rationalizations, Recognized, Analyzed and Ultimate Destroyed*!

What made me realize I needed to lose weight was that one day I got out of the shower, and, I think for the first time in my life, I saw myself as I was, and I panicked. I was disgusted with what I was looking at; you see, I was in denial for so many years as my physique was concerned.

"Who is that fat guy looking at me from the other end of that mirror? No that can't be me, no no."

It took me a week to sink in that I was fat, and it took me another week to figure out how I had managed to let myself reach to this sick and potentially life-threatening physique.

I cried; I am not going to lie. I was 36 years old, and I looked 55, not to mention my fitness level, where I was probably even more elderly.

What made me get off my fat ass was vanity, yes I admit it, I didn't start losing weight because I wanted to be healthy or because it was the right thing to do; no, it was straightforward and pure vanity. I wanted to return to that lean, mean, fit, sexy running machine I used to be in high school.

Well, if you read thus far, it means you already started to change your way of thinking, so let's start losing those pounds safely and healthy, and never gain them back.

Before we proceed, I need to say that I am not a doctor or have any medical training, so for any life-changing procedures you want to start, you should always consult your doctor or dietician, someone that has a medical diploma.

Ok, disclaimer out of the way, let's make the first step to a hopefully beautiful journey.

Weight Loss Tip Number 1 – Start walking

Unless you are 500 kilos and can't move, you can start walking right now as we speak. Stop giving excuses to yourself and get off that comfortable chair, relaxing couch or soft bed, and start walking. Before you start though, my advice is to get a physical from your doctor first. Tell him/her what you want to do so he/she will check you out thoroughly. A cardiograph is one of the things you should do; see how the old ticker is doing.

Always check with your doctor first when you are going to make major life changes, like exercise, new dietary lifestyles, new medicine, and everything that has to do with your health.

Walking is easy, it doesn't cost anything, just wear your sneakers or some athletic shoes. If you don't have any, don't worry, as you don't need them to just start walking.

Start slow, aim for a gradual increase in your workload. Do not walk every day, walk every two days instead, and gradually go to every other day and then every day.

It's in your hands, well actually, it's in your legs; nobody will walk for you.

Start with as much time you feel comfortable. I know some people suggest that you start with 5 minutes and then increase accordingly, but maybe for you is less than 5 minutes or maybe more.

Just get up your butt and walk. See how much time you can walk until it puffs you out;this would be your base. If you started walking, and, after 7 minutes, you started getting breathless, then that's your base!

Walk every two days for 7 minutes. When you see that you can do 7 minutes every two days with no difficulty, that means your fitness lever just went up. Now, start doing 7 minutes every other day, and apply the same philosophy. When you see that you can walk easily and without any effort for 7 minutes every other day, then go for 7 minutes every day and apply the same philosophy again.

When you see that 7 minutes every day has become a piece of cake for you, then increase the minutes walking until you reach your next level of breathless, find your new base, and apply the algorithm again.

I know I know I am too detailed in my description, but I need you to see that it's going to take time, and you need to do it gradually.

The most important thing to remember here is to take the decision and get out of the house or stay in the house if you have a trend mill.

From my experience, finding a friend to walk with is much helpful, and you increase your chances of sticking with the walking habit and turning it into a lifestyle.

Weight Loss Tip Number 2 – Walking and Running

At some point, you are going to be able to walk with ease and without any breathless point for 30 to 45 minutes, and that's when it will start to become a little bit boring.

Your body is going to start feeling the positive outcomes of your exercise, and it's going to start asking you for more.

You are going to feel the need for speed, and you are going to have this urge to keep up the pace and start running like crazy-like you are possessed or something. The truth is you are; you are possessed by this beautiful state of body and mind where, for the first time, after many years of idleness, you are rediscovering that you can accomplish things; it's the moment where you stopped being a "wisher" and become a "doer".

I mean, think about it a few weeks ago, you were just a couch potato, whereas now, you can walk 30 to 45 minutes without even breaking a sweat!

My advice if you feel the urge to go faster is to do just that, go faster, run like crazy, and enjoy the moment!

My wisdom here for you is not to go immediately from walking to running, that's not taking it easy. Your body just started getting into shape but needs a long way yet to be in the fitness state that will allow you to become a runner. Instead, do what I did, for about 2 to 3 months- let's call it transition period - I would walk and run alternatively for 30 to 45 minutes increasing the time gradually until I reached to 90 minutes to 2 hours.

Every person is different; he or she may decide to do more than what I did or less, it doesn't matter. Listen to your body and plan and act accordingly.

So very important to go through this transition period where you will combine walking and running. It will make you even stronger physically, it will increase your fitness level slowly and gradually, giving enough time to your body to cope with the physical stress you put on it and also the changes you see will be long-term and lasting.

Your self-esteem and self-confidence will go up and improve immensely, and, by doing this transitional phase, you eliminate the risk of getting disappointed because you didn't do so well with just pure running.

This is exactly what I would want you to avoid with this transitional period. If you go from walking to running without the transition, you will risk going too fast too hard, getting either your body or your psyche injured (getting depressed or disappointed). The reason is that your body will not be ready to produce the workload your emotional state will be asking because your physical state will not be ready yet to deliver.

Weight Loss Tip Number 3 –Running baby, yes! Oh yes!

If you stick with the walking and also go through the transition period that I am proposing (walking and running at the same time), then your body will be in a good physical place. I am sure you will notice some weight loss and, most importantly, your mood will be better; you will feel more happy, more satisfied, more optimistic, your depression will start to wear off and be replaced by your self-esteem and confidence, which are going to be high up. Generally, you will feel there is nothing you can't do as long as you set it as a goal, apply proper time management and go execute it.

Congratulations if you have followed my advice and felt all or some of the things I just described! You are starting to think and feel like a winner instead of a loser. This is the psychological state you need to be in, which will enable you to make the drastic changes necessary for you to change your mindset first, and, as a result, change your body as well.

Now, a few pieces of advice about running. You will follow the same tactic as you did with walking. First, go pay your doctor a visit and get a physical. Tell him/her you intend to start running as a way to become fitter and also lose weight, and he/she will give you the tests needed. Make a cardiograph again, and I am sure you will see some improvements in your heart rate, not much but noticeable. If I were a gambler, which I am not, I would bet your heart rate went down a few beats!

If you went through the transition period, then you will know your base for running, meaning how much time you can run comfortable without gasping for air.

Try and run 3 to 4 days a week. Do not - I repeat –do NOT run every day, do not make the same mistake I did when I first started running, assuming that a day without running is a lost one. NO, it's not like that, resting days are equally(if not more) important than running days.

3 to 4 days a week running. Start with the base you have and gradually increase the minutes or the mileage. There is a 10% rule, which goes roughly like this: if you did – let's say - 2 hours of running the first week, then the next weekit's going to be 2 hours plus 10% of the two hours, which equals to 2 hours and 12 minutes of running. The third week run 2 hours and 12 minutes plus 10%, which is 13 minutes, and so on.

If you want to learn more about how to train and finish your first 5k race, you can always check out my book with the same title. Subscribe to my mailing list, and you can have it as a gift! That's how much I want to help you that I'm giving away one of my books. I want you to understand that exercise, and especially running, will help you lose weight and change that metabolism of yours. Also, you can check out my post (put the link about the free plans in the freebies section)

You maybe needing a good pair of running shoes now and maybe invest in some running gear too. A visit online and also in the running section of my blog will give you enough information about what you should be looking for.

The secret is to embrace running as a way of life. Do it on your own time, own pace and own leisure. Do not force yourself to do anything that you don't like. Running or any other kind of exercise you decide to practice should be a way of releasing stress, and also a way of relaxing, and it should be a period of time where you are enjoying yourself.

Weight Loss Tip Number 4 –Eat lots of small meals during the day.

When you start walking, and later running or doing any other kind of exercise, your body is going to be forced to deliver more energy that it was used to deliver so far. It's going to need more fuel. Now, a lot of you will think, "why should I eat more? If I eat more, how am I supposed to lose weight?"

It's a valid question, but what we want to achieve with running is to start poking that slow metabolism of yours to start doing that which it is supposed to do, metabolize.

By running, you burn calories. Some of them come from fat, some others from carbs, while some of them are from protein. It is good to burn calories; burning calories means you lose weight, but it's important to eat many meals and snacks during the day. This way you are "confusing" your metabolism, and it doesn't know when you are going to feed it next, so you are messing up with its routine. I mean your body is not stupid; if you got it used to receive three big meals at specific times in the day, it's not going to burn any calories because it knows that John or Jane is going to feed me at 8 a. m. , 1 p. m. , and 8 p. m. for example.

Now, by eating at least 6 small meals during the day, you are messing up its timetable, and it doesn't know what to do. So, except for the fact that it burns more energy now to digest those 6 meals a day, it also starts to burn calories because it doesn't know when you are going to feed it again.

Plus, most important of all, eating small nutrient-dense meals throughout the day keeps you full, satisfied, and you don't end up binging on junk food at the end of the day and close to sleep time.

So, start applying having at least 6 small meals a day. Be careful not to starve yourself though because it will have the exact opposite result.

If you don't give your body the calories it needs, then the body will go into starvation mode. When the body is in that mode, it assumes that it will not receive food for a long period of time and, instead of burning calories, it starts to store calories, turning them into fat, and burn a very small amount of them.

So, do not starve yourself, eat small meals, but they should be filling. The ideal will be to take the same amount of calories you took when you had your three meals a day, but now you will be getting them with 6 meals a day.

You need to experiment a little with your food and see how it goes, every person is unique, and you are the only one that can figure this out. Of course, you can always visit a dietician who is more than able to help you with this.

Weight Loss Tip Number 5 – Drink water the moment you wake up.

A big chunk of headaches, migraines, some pains and other chronic conditions exist because, in our majority, we don't drink water at all. We are a society that is chronically dehydrated.

We are 60 to 70% water as body mass is concerned, and on a cellular level, we are 90%!!! When I found out this small piece of information, it just hit me, we need to drink water, people!

I used to assume that when peeing yellow or dark orange urine that it was natural and that my kidneys were actually working fine! How ignorant was I! When your urine is yellow or dark yellow you are severely dehydrated, and you need to drink a LOT of water.

People, if you want to lose weight, start drinking water at least 2 liters a day. The best time to drink water is right after you wake up in the morning, on an empty stomach. Just drink half a liter down, give your body a chance to hydrate after a long time of being dehydrated during sleep.

Yes, when we sleep the body tries to repair itself, it gets rid of toxins and a zillion other impurities, and it does that by using water.

By drinking water, you are making your blood thinner, and it flows better and more efficiently through your body, feeding your cells faster and also removing toxins and waste from the cells quicker.

Water helps you have better and easier bowel movements and a lot of your weight, a lot of pounds actually are a waste. This waste is stacked on the walls of your big intestines, and it is just rotting there, reintroducing toxins back into your bloodstream.

By drinking lots of water and with every successful bowel movement, you will see that all that waste will gradually start to get out, you will feel lighter, and also you will notice considerable weight loss.

Now, if you exercise and you run in hot weather, it's important to supplement with electrolytes. Ask your doctor or your chemist about what kind are best and when to take them.

You need to replenish your electrolytes, especially after a hard, sweaty running.

So, drink lots of water, aim for two liters at least, it will help you detoxify faster, and you need to embrace this practice of drinking water as a lifestyle.

Drink your water in a fun enjoyable way; don't see it as a chore that you need to do.

Let me give you an example: When I wake up in the morning, I go immediately and drink 2 glasses of water, total of about 500 ml, and I have my supplements with that.

When I reach the office, I drink another two glasses, that's another 500 ml of water, so by 7:30 a. m. I've already drunk 1 liter of water, and I am feeling refreshed and awake.

Then, I drink the rest of the water gradually through the day.

My work colleague has another system that works for him: He has bought a 2-liter bottle. The first thing he does when he comes to work is to fill that bottle with water and set it on his desk. By having it in front of him, he remembers he must drink water, and by the time he leaves work, he makes sure he has drunk all of it.

I just gave you two examples of two different people doing two different things as water consumption is concerned. Some of you might do the same thing like my colleague or like me, and I am sure there are others who have other ways and means to drink their quota of water. The important thing here is to remember that you need to start hydrating yourself. It will make you healthier, and you will see your skin starting to clear up and become younger. You will also flush all those toxins and waste out faster, you will clean your big intestine from all that waste that is stacked there, and you will see noticeable weight loss, as long as you adopt drinking water as a lifestyle habit.

Weight Loss Tip Number 6 – Finish eating at least 2 hours before bed time.

When we wake up as I mentioned in the previous tip, it is paramount to drink as much water as we can because, during the night, the body is repairing itself and also fighting illnesses using water, which results in us waking up dehydrated.

When we wake up, the first light of the sun notifies our brain that it's time to wake up, and a surge of energy is filling our body. We are more energetic in the early hours of the day, and as we go towards nightfall, our energy levels drop because our body is getting prepared to go to sleep. So, it will repeat the cycle of repair, heal, fight off invaders and rest, so the next morning, you will be able to have a healthy and energized day.

The last thing the body needs from you, just before you go to bed, is to assign it another job, which also happens to be one of the most energy required ones, digestion.

Think for a moment the following information, 10% of the calories we eat is used by the body to perform the digestion! 10% is a lot of calories and a lot of load for the body.

There are people that after they eat they literally stop doing anything. They just sit like zombies on a chair or lie on a bed because the energy that is required for the digestion makes them numb and can't move. Of course, that means they eat a lot, and they eat the wrong kind of food, but nevertheless, energy consumption for the completion of digestion is huge enough as it is, and it's something that you do not want to assign to your body right when is bedtime.

Because if you eat and then after 10 minutes you go to bed, first you will have weird dreams and sometimes nightmares. The whole unnatural process you put your body through sometimes manifests like that. Second, the body will not be able to complete the repairs, the healing process, and the rest process because instead of using energy to do that, it will use that energy to digest the food you just ate.

Your last meal should be 2 to 3 hours before the time you intend to sleep. If you get hungry, let's say an hour or 30 minutes before your planned bedtime, drink some water because you maybe feeling thirsty and not hungry. If that does not help, then eat something that can be easily digested in 30 minutes, like any kind of fruit, much better, seasoned fruits.

Do not - I repeat - do not consume refined or processed or even unprocessed food 30 minutes before you go to bed or 10 minutes before you go to bed.

Train yourself to eat 6 times a day. Eat light health-dense food and you will see that you won't have food cravings at night, and even if you do, they will not be as severe, and you can get away with it with a few fruits.

Weight Loss Tip Number 7 – Drink water 30 minutes before having a meal.

When we put food in our mouth, the process of digestion starts. Yes, digestion starts from the mouth, the mouth detects what kind of food we are eating, carbs or fat, and through the saliva, it secretes the appropriate enzymes to aid the digestion. So, the mouth also helps the digestion by chewing the food well. Then, when the food is chewed well, preferably until it becomes a soup-like context, it goes through the esophagus to the stomach and there the stomach produces hydrochloric acid. This very powerful acid turns the food into liquid even more, so when it reaches the small intestine, it will be much more easily for the nutrients to pass through the small intestine'svery thin walls.

When you drink water while eating or right after food, what you achieve is to disturb and obstruct the normal procedure of digestion by diluting the hydrochloric acid, making it weaker, thus, not liquefying the food ingredients correctly, thus making the job of the small intestine harder. And sometimes nutrients do not get absorbed because the weak acid cannot do its job properly.

So, make sure you drink water 30 minutes before you eat. By the time you eat, the water will have left the stomach. Therefore, It will not weaken the peptic acids.

Also, drink water 2 to 3 hours after you eat for the exact same reason.

Just try it and you will see tremendous changes in the way your digestive system will behave.

Weight Loss Tip Number 8 – Never eat fruit after a meal containing carbs or meat.

Fruits are mostly water, so treat fruits like water and apply the rules I mentioned in the previous tips. Eat fruits on an empty stomach, especially watermelon and melon; they are about 90% water anyway.

Eat fruits 30 to 45 minutes before your main meals and never right after a meal that has a combination of other foods.

Fruits get digested fast, and specific enzymes are used. Plus, fruits help us preserve our stored enzymes because they come packed with their own enzymes already.

If you eat fruits right after a big meal, then you run the risk of getting indigestion, heartburn, burping and other digestive discomforts. The reason for this is that the fruits are held in the stomach too long along with the other foods, and as a result, they rot and ferment in the gut, giving you an upset stomach. If you let it uncontrolled, it could lead to other health problems that derive from the digestive system.

Be smart; eat and then have your fruits after 2 to 3 hours, or 30 to 45 minutes before your main meals.

By having fruits before your main meal, will probably help you to eat less of your main meal, thus, assist you with your weight loss and weight control. Fruits are full of fibers which keep you satisfied longer.

Just try and see if there is any difference; have a meal one day, and then on another day have the same meal but have the fruits before (30 to 45 minutes).

Weight Loss Tip Number 9 – Apply mono-food eating.

Mono what? Well, mono in Greek means 'only one thing', so by eating only one type of food in every meal, you don't make your body produce a variety of enzymes but only a specific set that is ruined for the specific food you will eat.

For example, when you are eating fava beans, eat just fava beans; do not eat anything else but fava beans. This is the principle behind it.

The more complex and more varied a meal is, the more enzymes are produced and the more time the digestion needs, with all the side-effects that this may bring, such as bloating, swelling, heartburn, etc.

I always try to keep my meals on one or two, sometimes three ingredients at most, and I noticed that my digestion is faster, without any bloating or gas anymore.

Of course, you can combine lots of different food that belong to the same family.

For example, you can eat a big green vegetable salad because all the ingredients need pretty much the same enzymes.

The secret is to experiment and see what works for you.

Weight Loss Tip Number 10 – Water fast at least once a week.

I usually water fast every Friday for many reasons, it's the last working day for me and weekend comes so I can sleep in a bit more after I water fast to help my body get the needed rest.

The reason that I water fast is because of the calorie restriction you accomplish with it.

Research and studies have shown that when you restrict calories in living beings, their life expectancy increases.

So, what's one day compared to the opportunity to increase your life even for a few more years?

Second reason I water fast is that when you drink only water, you are giving a necessary and needed rest to your digestive system.

The third reason is that the body sees this as an opportunity, instead of spending time and energy on the consumption, digestion, and elimination of food, to spend that energy on repairing, healing, and fighting off viruses and bacteria.

By giving your body waterfast, you allow your immune system to work faster, better and deeper.

By drinking only water, you allow your blood to be diluted, making the flow of it to all of your organs and cells faster. This, in turn, will remove the waste and the toxins faster, and also it will feed your cells better using your fat deposits and glycogen deposits of the liver.

Weight Loss Tip Number 11 – Colon cleansing at least every two months.

Yes, you heard right. Colon enemas are the best way to clean all that waste that is stacked and petrified on the walls of your big intestine.

The reason most people suffer from constipation, hemorrhoids, bad acne and a series of other skin diseases and infections is that our big intestine is not clean.

Trust me, I know. I had chronic constipation, and you can imagine how hard it was also dealing with my hemorrhoids ;it was like excreting glass! I wish nobody will feel the pain I felt.

There are 4 kinds of enemas you can do, you can always get advice from doctors and medical care personnel on how to administrate one by yourself.

I started with distilled water because distilled water doesn't have any metals in it; it'spure, and it's clean.

I inject as many enemas as needed just with water until I see that my colon is clean enough.

After that, I administrate coffee enemas. I use organic grinded coffee beans and also distilled water. I boil the coffee for about 15 minutes until most of the coffee oils evaporate and then I wait for it to cool down until my finger can stand the temperature.

Then, I administrate the coffee and try to keep it in my big intestine for 15 minutes. I lie on my right side because the caffeine has better chances of getting absorbed by the haemorrhoidal veins of the colon. Caffeine is a stimulant and aids our liver to release toxins. Coffee enemas are not to help elimination.

So, first, I do a couple of water enemas, clean my colon well, and then a coffee enema to help my liver to get rid of toxins.

Weight Loss Tip Number 12 – Replace white sugar with brown sugar.

Easier said than done, many will say. Well, for me white processed sugar was one of the last nutritional culprits I stopped eating. It is addictive, I know the feeling. I was a heavy drinker of sodas from high school until I was diagnosed with a stomach ulcer, and I stopped all caffeinated drinks altogether.

Even after I stopped eating meat and dairy products, I would still indulge myself in sweats made out of white sugar.

Managing to stay away from was a matter of time until I figured out how to replace those empty calories with something more nutritional like, for example, blackstrap molasses or dates which have the sweetness of the white sugar but are not empty calories; they are packed with natural sugar, glucose and also minerals like calcium, iron and many more.

If you are making your own sweets try and replace white with brown, brown is the lesser evil, or try to use stevia another sweetener that has no calories at all. Stevia is excellent to use in your coffee or tea. It'ssweet but has no calories at all, how cool is that?!

Other sweeteners you can use is Maple Syrup and Agave nectar. I swear Agave nectar tastes like honey. Nutritional-wise, both of them are not that great; they are just sweeteners, but hey, all of the things I mentioned are sure much healthier comparing to the white devil.

Whenever you have your sweet teeth coming, eat some fruits, or make a fruit salad and put some maple syrup on top.

The sugar (fructose and glucose) that fruits contain are our natural sugar that our body is designed to use and absorb efficiently, and because fruits contain fiber, the glucose is slowly released into your blood stream, keeping us full and not hungry for a longer period of time.

White sugar is refined and processed, lacks fiber, and is not designed for our body. It gives a sudden boost of energy and then it's gone, and we need to eat again and again many times to maintain a level of fullness, but, at the same time, consuming empty calories that turn into fat.

Try and gradually replace white sugar, stay away from sugary sodas, refined and processed juices that are full of stuff. Make your own juices, invest in a juicer.

Weight Loss Tip Number 13 – Replace white flour with whole wheat flour.

Stay away from white flour. White flour is so refined and processed that it lacks fiber, one of the most important dietary agents we must aim to consume as much as possible daily. We evolved actually to consume up to 100grams of fiber daily!

The consumption of so much fiber every day enable the body to dump a lot of toxins in our colon which then would get eliminated through defecation.

Bread and other products that are made out of white flower lack fiber and they are also again like white sugar; empty calories with no nutritional value only making you more fat.

Prefer products that are made from whole wheat or another kind of whole flour. They have fiber, and their nutritional value is superior to white flour products.

Brown bread is much better than white bread. Try it, you have nothing to lose, only to gain your health back.

Weight Loss Tip Number 14 – Replace White Salt with Pink Salt or Low Sodium Salt.

Do not be fooled. High salt intake is responsible for a range of illnesses and conditions like gastric cancer, recurrent kidney stones, osteoporosis, obesity, and direct renal vascular and cardiac damage.

The grand prize though goes to high blood pressure. There is no debate, people, if white salt is good or bad for you;of course, it's bad for you; it has too much sodium and is killing you.

If you read articles that say low sodium diets are bad for you, check the author and find out if he or she works for the salt industry, who probably does.

There are hundreds of research and trials out there that show in black and white that white salt is harmful to our health.

I stopped using it anymore. I use either herbal salts with low sodium or Himalayan salt (always organic), or I use a lot of celery in my cooking, which is packed with natural sodium.

Weight Loss Tip Number 15 – Replace animal milk with plant based milk

I have written extensively about how bad animal milk is for us. I feel like I am repeating myself by saying this, but it's the truth, and I will repeat this information until everybody on this planet get the following statement(I am sorry about the cap letters, but it's a way to emphasize the importance): THE MILK OF ANOTHER ANIMAL IS NOT HEALTHY FOR HUMAN CONSUMPTION. There, I said it, and I got it out of my system.

The only milk that is appropriate for our DNA is our mother's milk, which is suitable for our genetic code and had the right analogies of protein, carbs and fat, and numerous other beneficial nutrients for us.

Until our mother stops breastfeeding us, the ideal is to be breastfed until 2 years old, yes, you heard right, that's the ideal time.

If a mother breastfeeds her baby for two years, the offspring has better chances of survival and also no PMS for the ladies; as long as you breastfeed you don't have any new eggs because it's a defense mechanism that prevents you from staying pregnant while you are taking care of your baby.

So, after we have been cut out from mommy's milk, sorry about the caps again, WE DO NOT NEED ANY MORE MILK EVER AGAIN. Ahh, that felt good again!

Animal milk does not help you have strong bones, it actually makes exactly the opposite, it aids along with other factors to give you osteoporosis and brittle bones, yes you heard right again. So, stop drinking animal milk, you are destroying your bones.

There are so many other sources of where you can get your calcium, much better absorbable than the calcium in animal milk.

(Name a few here)

Try new plant-based milk. There are many types out there, like soy milk, or almond milk, which is my favorite, and you can totally prepare it at home. (Describe here how to make almond milk)

Weight Loss Tip Number 16 – Replace white rice with brown rice.

You may now ask why. All the Chinese are eating white rice. Yes, so? Just because they eat it, doesn't mean it's good for you.

White rice is the remaining starch that was left from brown rice that had its shell removed. The shell, ladies and gentlemen, has the fiber that helps us feel fuller for a longer time, contributes in our bowel movements and is packed with a variety of B vitamins.

Years ago, when the greedy merchants of the past discovered that if they removed the shell of the brown rice, they could increase the shelf time of rice, they started applying it in bulk. It was when people started to die like flies that they realized that something wrong was happening.

By removing the hull of the brown rice and leaving only the starch substance, which is the white rice, they removed away the B vitamins, and people were dying from B complex Vitamin deficiency!

So, now what they do is that they take the brown rice, remove the hull, take the starch, which is the white rice, and add B vitamins to it! Crazy? Well, greedy business will do anything for money.

You don't have to be part of this greedy business. Buy brown rice, buy black rice, buy wild rice; sure it takes longer to cook, but at least it won't give you obesity!

Go brown, it is healthier. So, what if it lasts only 1 year on the shelf and not 4, like white rice? Please do the right thing for your health.

Weight Loss Tip Number 17 – Eliminate oils from your diet.

Oils, either they come from animals or plants, are not good for you. They are highly refined and processed, and they offer nothing as nutritional value is concerned. Yes, even olive oil. Stay away from them, they are almost 100% fat. The soonest they enter your body, the body doesn't use them at all; it just adds them to your fat deposits.

There are many other ways of cooking or preparing sweets or other cakes without using oils.

Fried cooking is bad for you and doesn't offer you anything nutrition-wise. The oils increase the calorie count of the food exponentially, giving you "empty" calories.

A nice example is the potatoes. If you eat boiled potatoes, you can eat as much as you want and never worry that you get fat; they are low in calories and are filling, especially if you cook them with their skin.

Now, if you take the same quantity of potatoes and fry them, you have a bomb of "empty" calories, meaning only fat and no nutritional value for you. You will be eating the same quantity, but frying potatoes will add chemicals to your food that are carcinogen in nature, let alone that their calories will be ten times the calories of the original potatoes.

Weight Loss Tip Number 18 – Replace Processed Carbs with natural ones.

People make a lot of mistakes as nutrition is concerned, fatal mistakes. I used to be one of them. Now, I want to believe that I don't make the same mistakes of the past, sure I am still making mistakes, but at least adopting a whole plant-based diet for the last three years is not lethal as my previous nutritional lifestyle was (animal products and a lot of refined and processed carbohydrates).

Refined carbohydrates give a bad name to carbohydrates. You will see a lot of diets out there named low carb diets, which are dangerous for your health, and you should never follow them.

The whole plant-based unrefined and unprocessed carbohydrates, either simple, like fruits or complex, like legumes and starch, are the natural food of the human body. The only thing they promote is a healthy way of living because they help you lose weight or maintain your existing weight and also provide all the essential minerals, vitamins, fiber and antioxidants the body needs to be able to have an optimum level of working efficiency. Animal products and processed carbohydrates, like white sugar, white rice, white flour, sweets prepared with animal or plant-based oils, or white sugar and heavily processed oils, like corn oil, are all devoid of nutrients, minerals, and vitamins. Their antioxidant levels are low, fiber is almost absent, and they are "empty" calories; they just fill your stomach, but they don't feed your body.

I will give you three basic examples, so you understand what I am talking about. Prefer to eat 3 to 4 red juicy apples with some Ceylon cinnamon on top instead of eating an apple pie that's made of white sugar, eggs, and refined oils. The apple in that pie, nutritionally speaking, is dead; it's just weight and empty calories. It's filled with fat, eggs and oils that are not good for you (saturated), fats that will clog your arteries and white sugar that will spike your insulin levels, resulting in the accumulation of more fat and the temporary boost of energy.

On the other hand, 3 to 4 apples will give you energy that lasts for at least 2 hours or more because they have the natural sugars the body knows how to use and utilize, such as glucose and fructose. These natural sugars can be easily transformed into glycogen, the fuel of the human body.

Second example: Prefer to eat olives, either black or green, instead of putting olive oil in your salads, using it to cook or using it to eat your legumes and other food.

Olives have fiber, minerals, vitamins and are not highly processed as olive oil, which is basically almost 100% fat, and which the body doesn't really know how to use or process. It just stores it in your fat deposits.

Third example: Prefer to make your own juice of oranges or your own smoothie instead of drinking packaged juices that are filled with artificial colorings, preservatives, and white sugar.

I think I made my point.

Weight Loss Tip Number 19 – Gradually reduce your meat consumption.

I know a lot of you are rolling your eyes right now, but I know exactly how you feel, I used to roll my eyes too when 4 or 5 years ago I would read articles about a plant-based diet.

I was not a heavy meat eater from the age of 35 until 38 when I stopped eating animal products, but I had been eating a lot of meat and especially red and processed meat from the age of 20 until 35.

I know now that meat and dairy consumption are the reasons that at the age of 30 I was diagnosed with a series of digestive track illnesses, like esophagus ulcer, stomach and duodenum ulcer, hemorrhoids, constipation and heart burns.

I describe my "Odyssey" in my first book, *Thirsty for health* in great detail.

As I said in my book, I was glad that my body gave in and couldn't take any more abuse by the meat consumption because it made me alert as to start searching what's wrong with me.

When I gradually started to eliminate my meat intake and also started applying an exercise regime, mostly running, I became a new man. All the above diseases that I mentioned do not exist anymore, and also I lost 44 pounds safely and never gained them back as I describe in my book *My weight loss Journey. . .*

Society is led to believe that to get some protein you need to eat meat and to get your calcium you need to drink animal milk.

The two above assumptions that today are considered to be facts by millions of people are just that, assumptions.

Yes, you get protein by eating the flesh of dead animals, but you can also get more than enough of the amino acids that the body cannot produce from a balanced, whole grain, plant-based diet.

Plus, our body has amino acids stores. For someone to become protein deficient, he or she must starve to death like the unfortunate kids in Africa and other parts of the world where starvation is a daily situation.

You don't need milk coming from animals and especially cow's milk to get your calcium. You can also get your calcium from a whole grain, plant-based diet and it's more absorbable than milk calcium. (Find plant-based calcium sources and write them here)

Let's assume that you eat meat, that you want to get protein, why would you risk getting cholesterol and saturated fat, both substances that are proven to be the culprits of heart diseases, stroke, diabetes 2, high blood pressure, high cholesterol, and a series of more severe illnesses?

Why would you continue to drink milk –cow's milk – when it's proven and shown that it only makes your bones more brittle and gives you osteoporosis?

Why not adopt gradually a whole grain, unprocessed plant-based diet and lifestyle that you can get your protein and your calcium from, minus all the "bad guys" –cholesterol and saturated fat?

Weight Loss Tip Number 20 – Gradually reduce sodas and sugary drinks from your diet.

When we were kids my parents could only afford to buy us food and clothes, so we didn't have sugary products in the house like chocolates, colas and various types of sodas. We had some, but not the phenomenon you see these days where kids are gulping down a huge amount of sugary drinks like there is no tomorrow.

I used to drink Coke with a vengeance until I was 31 years old where I was diagnosed with a stomach ulcer and that was for caffeinated drinks. I went cold turkey and never put them in my mouth again.

When you are hooked to these empty-calorie, promoting-obesity liquids, you don't feel how sweet they are.

Do this experiment, stay away from them for a month and then go try and drink one of this fizzy drinks; I promise you, you will want to throw up, that's how much sugar they have.

Soda is very acidic; it's only one point higher on the pH scale than battery acid! Thus, it is terrible for people who suffer from acid reflux.

With each can of soda, you get about 150 calories, which are empty calories because you don't feel any fuller and they are not nutritious. Caffeinated soda, which was my soda of choice, has between 30 to 55 mg of caffeine, and is also loaded with sulphites, artificial coloring, and dangerous high fructose corn syrup.

Do you know how many teaspoons of sugar a can of soda has? On average, a can of soda contains ten teaspoons of the "white devil". Every time you drink a can of soda, you are putting ten teaspoons of refined white sugar into your body. The phosphoric acid is added to soft drinks to give them a sharper flavor. Phosphoric acid can interfere with the body's ability to use calcium; chronic consumption of sodas may lead to osteoporosis.

Weight Loss Tip Number 21 – Gradually reduce and eliminate coffee from your diet.

I know I know you are rolling your eyes again. "I can't live without coffee" and statements like that. Well, I am the living proof that you CAN live without coffee. Don't get me wrong, you can use coffee in other applications, just don't drink it.

It's a stimulant that, over time, it wears out the nervous system, and our adrenal glands get fatigued of producing hormones on demand so you can go through the day.

Caffeine is addictive, and, like nicotine, it creates a dependency. You don't need stimulants to function; what you need is a healthy plant-based lifestyle with enough exercise and adequate sleep.

There are a lot of studies about coffee, conflicting each other. Of course, like all big industries (meat, egg, dairy, pharmaceutical, tobacco), the coffee industry is paying scientists to tell their version of truth, even when the scientific data do not support them.

Just think that it took 7000 studies to prove beyond reasonable doubt that smoking kills, before the Surgeon General of the USA came out in 1964 and admitted the obvious, that smoking kills.

It's the same think with meat; meat today is the new smoking. It will take some time to get the whole truth out.

I am not saying that coffee kills, like smoking does, or meat consumption, but why consume something that makes your liver work overtime to get rid of it?

One of the things that led to me kicking my caffeine habit was being diagnosed with an ulcer (which was worsened by caffeine consumption and smoking). I did not stop the coffee and soda drinking cold turkey; I was too hooked to stop like that, so I stopped like the waves of the sea. At the beach, you see the waves coming; sometimes you see a big wave that hits the shore, and then a second one with the same form and grace but with less intensity, and then a third comes with the same characteristics but with even less intensity, until there are no waves left.

So one day, I sat down and calculated how many milligrams of caffeine I was consuming a day. It was more than 600 mg a day, which is too much. I created an 8-week program to gradually cut back on caffeine; I reduced my caffeine intake by 100 mg per week until I spent the final weeks without any caffeine.

While this method lessened the withdrawal effects, I still experienced caffeine withdrawal (albeit in a milder form and to a smaller degree of intensity). I used to have cellulite—yes, guys can have it; it's not just a woman thing—but after I stopped consuming caffeine and increased my water volume, it disappeared.

Why are adults so careful not to let their kids consume any caffeinated products because of the negative side effects, yet, as adults, they all drink coffee together as a family? People don't think about it; they just begin their caffeine dependency and only consider changing when medical problems start to appear.

The same goes for other things in life: we are so careful to ensure that our children are healthy, yet we neglect our own health, and as soon as our children are grown up, a healthy lifestyle is generally abandoned.

I want to close this chapter with a sin I indulge in once a year: whenever I go to Bucharest to run the half-marathon there, a day before the race (always around noon), I have a small espresso. I never drink it in the cafeteria; I always drink it in my hotel room, because after I drink it, seconds later I get so high and dizzy that I can't stay up.

I lie on my bed and enjoy the caffeine buzz. That's how much caffeine affects me now; I can sense all its addictive effect because I am not desensitized to it anymore.

So, yes, every year I drink my espresso and I get my caffeine high. Try it. Stop drinking any coffee or caffeinated drinks or other products for a year and then have a small coffee, and you will understand completely what I mean.

Weight Loss Tip Number 22 – Breathing exercises.

Yes, you read right, breathing exercises will help you lose weight. How? Well, let me explain.

Most people on this planet suffer from two main simple conditions, they are chronically dehydrated, and they are chronically under oxygenated. This last condition is called hypoxia, meaning we do not give the necessary oxygen primarily to our brain and then to the rest of our body to be able to function as it should.

Many reasons lead to hypoxia, for example, smoking: people that smoke receive more carbon monoxide into their brain than oxygen or the air we breathe around us, especially in the big cities, is not that clean. Another reason can be when working for hours in air-conditioned places and so on.

The most important reason that we don't get enough oxygen is that we don't exercise. When you exercise, you are training your lungs to take more oxygen in and also making them more efficient to remove carbon dioxide out of your system.

By doing a few yoga-like breathing exercises every day, you achieve two things. First, relaxing from the stress of everyday life, and second, strengthening your lungs and making them more efficient to deliver oxygen to your body.

This is a lovely article by Bex that shows how benefit Yoga is for you.

http://twinsintrainers.com/finding-time-meditation/

Weight Loss Tip Number 23– Stop watching TV.

Now, how on earth stopping watching TV is going to help you lose weight? Well, let me tell you how.

Have you ever thought of how many hours you lose each day, sitting on your comfortable couch or chair and watching other people live their life? One hour? Two hours? Three hours? Four Hours?!!! Are you serious? Don't you see that by sitting on your butt all day, eating pizzas, and drinking beers or fizzy drinks you are not going to make that fat go away?

Stop watching TV! Yes, you can use the time that you are wasting on this activity to start a walking program and gradually turn it into a running training program. Nothing is impossible.

Now, stop crying like a little baby and hiding behind excuses, "oh, I don't have time to go exercise" or "I don't have time to do that. " STOP watching TV and get your butt out of that chair and start taking your life back. I just found you a LOT of time to do something, so stop hiding behind the I-DON'T-have-time excuse.

Weight Loss Tip Number 24– Stop Wasting your time with Social Media.

Yes, I am cutting that too. Who gives a dime of what kind of food you had for dinner or what the cat did in your living room? Stop wasting so much time on Facebook, Twitter or all those so-called social media which the last thing they do is to provide a real social life.

Stop answering your email every 5 minutes. You should spend 20 minutes top every day on social media, no more.

I bet you spend hours Tweeting and Instagramming or whatever else you are using. Make some changes, sit down and calculate how much time you spend on these activities, and if it's more than 20 minutes, then you need to stop, period.

You can do so many other things on the time you waste on social media; you can start an athletic activity, like cycling, running, walking or whatever you feel fancy doing, you can go out and meet real people instead of talking to them through little miniature LCD screens.

You can start a weight-training program. You can go learn how to cook healthier, you can learn how to cook plant-based recipes. The list is endless, just stop wasting your time with social media. Minimize it to the least possible time and use the time to better yourself, make it stronger both physical and emotional, aim to educate yourself.

Weight Loss Tip Number 25– Start watching Nutritionfacts. org videos.

One of the many websites that had and still has a profound impact on my life is nutritionfacts. org run by Dr. Michael Greger MD. The doctor is amazing; his entire site is based on receiving donations, so he is not under the control of the grand from big companies, so he is unbiased. All the data on that site is free, and it's truthful. I 100% trust Dr. Greger, and he helped me immensely to see the light and the error in my ways.

Remember when I told you to stop watching TV and wasting time on social media, well, you can use some of that time to go to this site and educate yourself about nutrition.

Every time I wake up in the morning, while I am doing my morning bowel movement, I watch a couple of videos.

Also, if you are more of a traditional type, buy his book that he just released. It's full of goodies and life-saving information, including how to lose weight.

His book is entitled *How not to die*. That's a cool title by the way, and you can buy it from his webpage or amazon.com.

Just buy the book, it's an investment, plus you'll be helping the doc to keep his org status and continue to give his unbiased data and information to us for free.

Weight Loss Tip Number 26– Buy these Books.

This is a list of some of the nutrition related books that I read and that helped me lose 44 pounds over a period of 3 years and never gained them back.

1. *How not to die by Michael Greger, MD*
2. *Thrive by Brendan Brazier*
3. *Eat & run – Un unlikely journey to ultra marathon greatness by Scott Jurek*
4. China Study by T. Colin Campbell, PhD
5. *Dr. Dean Ornish's Program for Reversing Heart Disease: The Only System Scientifically Proven to Reverse Heart Disease Without Drugs or Surgery by Dr. Dean Ornish*
6. *The 80/10/10 Diet by Dr. Douglas N. Graham*

7. *Prevent and Reverse Heart Disease by Caldwell B. Esselstyn, Jr., MD*
8. *What to eat when you are pregnant and Vegetarian by Dr. Rana Conway*
9. *The Hippocrates Diet and Health Program by Ann Wingmore*
10. *The food Recolution by John Robbins*
11. *Vegan for Life by Jack Norris, RD and Virginia Messina, MPH, RD*
12. *Skinny Bitch by Rory Freedman and Kim Barnouin*
13. *Diet for a new America by John Robbins*
14. *Vegan for Her by Virginia Messina, MPH, RD*
15. *My weight Loss Journey: How I lost 44 pounds and never gained them back using a plant based diet.*

Weight Loss Tip Number 27– Download these free books.

This is a small list of very interesting nutrition books that are free and helped me a lot.

The Fast-5 Diet And The Fast-5 Lifestyle by Bert W. Herring's M.D.
Why Humans like Junk Food by Steven A. Witherly's PhD
My Weight Loss Story: How To Lose Weight Safely And Permanently. By Andreas Michaelides

Weight Loss Tip Number 28– Start learning from these doctors and dieticians.

Neal Barnard, M.D.

Web sites: http://www.nealbarnard.org and Physician's Committee for Responsible Medicine (PCRM)

Colin Campbell, M.D.

Website: T. Colin Campbell Center for Nutrition Studies http://nutritionstudies.org

Caldwell Esselstyn, M.D.

Website: http://www.dresselstyn.com

Joel Fuhrman, M.D.

Website: http://www.drfuhrman.com

Michael Greger, M.D.

Websites: http://www.veganmd.org and NutritionFacts.org

Michael Klaper, M.D.

Website: http://doctorklaper.com

John McDougall, M.D.

Website: http://www.drmcdougall.com

Dean Ornish, M.D.

The Web sites http://deanornish.com/ and Preventive Medicine Research Institute

Jack Norris RD

Website http://jacknorrisrd.com/

Virginia Messina

Website www.theveganrd.com/

Weight Loss Tip Number 29– Stop going to junk food restaurants.

Isn't it funny that we actually say this phrase to each other, "junk food. ""What did you have last night Pete?", "Oh, I was tired so I ordered some junk food!!!"

We know it is junk food we eat on a daily basis. You know something, when you eat junk, you become junk; you are what you eat and most accurately you are what you can absorb in the thin layers of your small intestine!

Stop eating junk food. I know it's difficult, but this kind of food is full of three things: FAT, SALT, and SUGAR.

They are empty, useless calories, and they make you FAT! Wake up, just stop putting JUNK food in your mouth and into your body; your body must be a temple you must respect. When you respect something, you do NOT throw junk at it.

Educate yourself from the list of doctors I gave you earlier; see how they replace the junk food with whole healthy nutritional alternatives, and you will see it's not that hard to do. Also, it's much cheaper in the long run. How? I'll tell you how. When you eat junk food, you will give yourself a series of fatal and deadly diseases that before they end you, they are going to torture you slowly and gradually. You will spend thousands of your hard-earned money on pills, drugs and medical procedures, which the only thing they do is just to treat the symptoms and not the cause. STOP EATING JUNK FOOD. Invest your money on clean, nutritional, whole, plant-based food and aim for organic if you can afford it. If you can't, then even conventionally grown fruit and vegetables are 100 times healthier than animal products or refined and processed food.

Wake up. We only have one life. Live it healthy and happy and pain-free. Do not become a slave to junk food because they seem to be cheaper now and because they are convenient, and they are in every corner of this planet. Say NO! Take your life and your diet back and away from junk food restaurants. YOU are in control of your food, not them.

Weight Loss Tip Number 30– Increase your fruit consumption.

Remember when I told you in a previous entry on this article to gradually eliminate meat from your diet? Well, I know a lot of you probably even terminated your internet browser from frustration when I suggested that, so I am going to give you a different alternative and another healthier also approach.

Do not reduce your meat consumption, but instead, increase your fruit consumption. Do you think you can do that?

I am pretty sure you don't eat many fruits because if you did, you probably wouldn't have any weight problems.

Let's for a moment forget all the amazing beneficial attributes that fruits have for our body (Antioxidants, vitamins, minerals, etc.) The one thing that fruits are packed a lot with is fiber and guess, my good people, what fiber does? Well, it does two main things. First, it fills you up and keeps you satiated longer hours, and second, it does that only with a fraction of the calories you would have consumed if you had meat instead.

For example, if you eat 4 medium-sized bananas, that's approximately 400 grams and about 320 calories. I am using bananas because they are one of the most calorie-dense fruits out there. If you do that, this little snack will keep you satisfied and full for at least two hours depending on your exercise level of course. The glucose and fructose in the fruit are slowly released into our body because of the fiber, keeping you full for longer periods of time.

Guess what you don't do when you fill full and satisfied for longer periods of time. Exactly, my good friends, you don't eat more food, you don't eat every single hour junk fast food like chocolates, sweets and other similar products packed with empty, useless calories that only fill your stomach but do not feed your body.

So, yes, try and so this. Start at night, 1 hour before you go to sleep. If you are hungry, do not eat potato chips or chocolates or any other kind of refined sugar product. Eat some fruits, see how you feel in the morning.

Weight Loss Tip Number 31– Increase your vegetable consumption.

The same principle that applies for fruits applies for vegetables too. They are also packed with antioxidants, vitamins, minerals, fiber, and also water.

By eating vegetables, namely lots of salads in your diet, you are satisfying yourself in three ways. First, you get your much-needed fiber and with combination with adequate water and exercise you make sure you have effective and easy bowel movements. When you eat veggies, you can say goodbye to constipation!

When you eat a lot of vegetables, the insoluble fiber that they contain acts like a cleaning broom for the colon, removing all the toxins that the body dumps there in an effort to get rid of them.

Also, extra cholesterol is dumped too into the colon, and the fiber is the one that removes it from our system.

Green vegetables especially are packed with chlorophyll, the green substance of the plants that has beneficial applications for our colon flora and also for our body in general. It cleans and cleanses the blood.

Try and have salads as side dishes, start with that and gradually proceed to have just salads for lunch or dinner. You will see tremendous health benefits in a few months if you start eating more vegetables and also fruits. You won't have eating cravings often because the fiber and the slow release of the natural sugars they contain keep you satiated for longer periods of time.

Weight Loss Tip Number 32– Increase your legume consumption.

Legumes have been the base of my nutrition for the last three years now. I get my amino acids that the body cannot make on its own, but needs to get them from food. It's a Myth that you need to combine certain foods to get the whole range of your needed amino acids.

You just need to incorporate as many different plant-based categories of food into your week, and you are fully covered.

I get the bulk of my iron from them also, especially kidney beans and lentils, and other beans, of course, are packed with iron. I always combine it with lots of lemon juice (Vitamin C), which increases the iron absorption rate by six-fold.

Another thing that I get is the incredible fiber they contain, . Legumes remove the toxins from my colon, keep me full longer, lower my cholesterol – not that I need it, all the food I eat does not contain any cholesterol anyway.

I will eat legumes at least 3 to 4 times a week. A typical week for me will be something like this: Monday lentils, Wednesday white beans, Friday mung beans, Sunday Giant beans in the oven. The following week: Tuesday, peas, Thursday fava beans with greens, Saturday kidney beans.

I usually eat my legume dish around 4:30 when I come back from work or later around 6 p. m. after I finish with my workouts, either running or weight lifting.

You can always accompany your legumes with salads. Trust me; add more legumes to your diet and you will start seeing considerable weight loss, and the cool thing about it is that you can eat as much as you want and still lose weight because they are nutrient-dense and also their calories are not that many, as you might thing. Natural carbohydrates that are contained in fruits, vegetable and legumes are not to be afraid. What you need to stay away from is refined and processed carbohydrates like white rice, sugar, flour, etc. Stay away from oils, either animal or plant originated.

Weight Loss Tip Number 33– Increase your Starch consumption.

Now, Starch is my second favorite food category after legumes because they enable me to sustain myself adequately as calories and nutritional value are concerned. I usually eat them for dinner.

I will usually boil potatoes, and I will add them to my green salad. Stay away from fried potatoes; those things are empty calories, super bombs. A boiled potato is filling and gives a huge number of nutrients, especially its skin, so don't remove the skin, people; 60% of the nutrients are on the skin and has very low calories per gram. Also, potatoes is a complete protein, meaning it contains all the essential amino acids, you can only eat potatoes for months and cover your protein intake easily, this is for my meathead friends out there who still insist that meat is the only way to get your protein from!

An entire nation was living on potatoes for years, namely Ireland.

Sometimes, I boil potatoes and create puree, add some garlic and other dry herbs...yummy! I have jacket potatoes in the oven and fill them with baked pinto beans! Yummy, yummy, yummy!

Another starch category is brown rice. As I mentioned earlier, stay away from white rice, especially if you want to lose weight, white rice is shown in studies to be promoting obesity.

The third category is corn, sweet corn. I can boil it in a casserole and eat it as is, or I can use corn seed for popcorn. I usually eat popcorn while watching a documentary or a movie! Yummy!

So, try and incorporate this three types of food. The starchy type was the basis for a lot of ancient civilizations, The Incas in Peru had the potatoes, and that's where the bulk of the thousands of varieties of potatoes comes from. The Aztecs and the American Indians had corn as their base of their diet. Have you ever had bread made from unrefined corn flour? Yummy!

For Chinese, the bulk of their diet still today is rice. Have you seen an obese Chinese person? Have you wondered why? Yes, because they eat a lot of rice.

Start adding and experimenting with potatoes, corn, and rice, and you will start to see changes in your waistline for sure.

Weight Loss Tip Number 34– Increase your nuts consumption.

Are you nuts? How many times we heard that phrase either in the movies or in reality when someone is referring to a person or a situation that he or she considers being crazy.

Well, I have good news for you, NUTS are good for you; they are packed with fiber, vitamins, minerals, antioxidants, all the good fatty acids, like omegas 3 and 6, and also polyunsaturated and unsaturated fats.

I usually have them with my oats at work around 1 p. m. I get my daily omega-3 doses from one tablespoon flax seeds, a big percentage of my calcium from sesame seeds, my selenium from Brazilian nuts, a portion of my iron from pumpkin seeds, and a range of other nutrients that these seeds provide for me.

Now, not all seeds are good for you. Stay away from, again, processed ones which are usually the ones that are drowned in salt, so stay away from salted seeds. Try to get unsalted organic seeds or, if you can't afford organic, prefer the unsalted kind.

Also, do not eat a lot, there is a reason seeds are safely tucked away under a layer of shells. Once again, technology enables us to remove nutshell easy and have them readily available for our consumption, which is not good. Eat them but sparingly.

In the old days, when people were eating nuts, they had to climb trees or spend a considerable time gathering them and then breaking them to eat them, spending a big chunk of energy and calories to do this.

Now, we sit on our couch watching TV and eating salted nuts, which is not very healthy! Get the picture?

So, add unsalted nuts in your diet, but do not overeat them. See nuts as a supplement to your diet.

Weight Loss Tip Number 35– Drink more smoothies.

Smoothies are an excellent way to provide your body fast and without a lot of energy-waste nutrients, and fiber. The reason we need to chew well our food is to break the fiber enough so the nutrients inside become more readily available.

Also, by chewing well, we are making the digestion easier and the stomach's job faster. Ifyoutake small bites, the stomach will not take that much of time to dissolve the food before pushing it to the small intestine. If you swallow big chunks of food, and this is what usually happens when instead of chewing we gulp our food down, then the stomach is going to have to work harder to break the food, and also it will take longer.

So, by having smoothies on a regular basis, we achieve a very important task; we give our digestive system a much-wanted break because a smoothie is already in a dissolved form, easily digestible, and it will not task the stomach with working hard, and the nutrients will get absorbed better and faster.

Weight Loss Tip Number 36– Get 8 hours of sleep.

Our society has three chronic conditions that are slowly killing us from inside out. First one is the lack of proper and adequate exercise, we ended up being couch potatoes; we sit in front of the stupid box, that's how I call a TV these days, watching other people living our lives, our desires, our fantasies, and dreams. We do this "stupid" thing, watching TV and eating empty calories from junk food simultaneously. NO wonder there is an obesity epidemic!!!

The second condition is that we don't drink water anymore, 60 to 70% of our body weight is water and 90% on a cellular level we are water. Water is life, water is our life, without water simply there is no life.

Chronically dehydrated, under functioned, we drink everything and anything except the much-needed water. We drink coffee and tea, and sodas, and refined and processed juices and anything else that is made from white sugar as its base except the life-giving water.

We are killing ourselves by dehydrating ourselves day in and day out. A big chunk of headaches and migraines is because the brain doesn't oxygenate well because the blood becomes so thick and slow that does not move easily and freely so as to deliver the oxygen to our brain and other tissues.

The third condition is the lack of sleep as people in our culture underestimate sleep. Sleep deprivation, chronic sleep deprivation is shown in scientific experiments and studies to contribute to obesity and also heart conditions.

Our body needs to sleep to assess what needs to be fixed, repaired or rejuvenated. It does that by being completely still and not wasting energy on anything else so the body will use that precious energy and those precious calories to find bugs and viruses and deal with them, fight them and kill them. This energy is also to repair organs and limbs, to get rid of toxins that we put into our bodies willingly or unwillingly.

So, my advice is to try and get 8 hours of sleep every day, continuously not periodically, try to be in bed by 9 to 9:30 p. m. , that's the time that we get the best out of our night sleep.

Weight Loss Tip Number 37– Keep a Food Diary.

If in the past or still until today you are keeping some kind of diary then you realize the importance of one. If you didn't keep one thus far, let me give you a few reasons of the advantages to keeping one.

Let's say today you had heavy diarrhea, and you don't remember what you ate a few days ago, or you do, but you don't know exactly how much you ate and where the food came from.

If you had a diary where you write everything in there, what you ate, what time you ate, how much you ate, how it made you feel after you ate it, then you could pinpoint the food that caused you to have diarrhea or the circumstances that contributed to it.

There are types of food that we are allergic to, there are types that are intolerable, while others make us feel gassy or feel like Superman.

Like I said many times in the past in my books and also in my article here on my blog, every person is unique, and you need to search and find what works for you, which food makes you feel good and which makes you feel great; a diary will accomplish that.

Also, by keeping track of what you eat and an estimation of the quantities, you can use online calorie calculators, like cronometer.com to have a general idea of the nutrients you are getting, such as minerals, vitamins, fatty acids, etc.

Trust me. Start keeping a food diary. It doesn't take long of your time, 10 minutes tops. Instead of watching commercials on TV for 10 minutes, use that time to write down what you ate, when you ate it, how much approximately you ate, how it made you feel, and also include what you drank. Do it at night, a few hours before you go to bed, make it into a ritual and whenever you feel bad or uncomfortable, see what you ate, and you will see how useful it will be.

You will find out if some food combinations are better for you or worse.

Begin slowly and gradually, start by just cataloging what you eat, just the names, then start to incorporate quantity and time you ate, and how it made you feel.

Weight Loss Tip Number 38– Keep an Exercise Diary.

The same principle that guides you to keep a food diary also applies here. By keeping an exercise diary, you will be able to track your performance. Also, the most important thing about keeping a diary like this is that it's a way to keep yourself accountable.

What I mean by that:If at some point, you get the blues, or you feel sad, or you feel you are not doing enough or achieving enough, you can also pick up the diary and see where were you when you first started in the physical, psychological, and emotional state. You will see that you managed A LOT, and that will give you courage and determination not to give up, not to quit the effort you started to become a better version of yourself. Both physically, with positive results on your health, and also emotionally, with positive results also in your personal life and social surroundings.

When you are a positive-thinking person, and all your thoughts and actions emit optimism, then this is transferred to your immediate social circle, and they, in their turn, also become optimists, emitting pleasant emotions that come back to you uplifting you even more. The saying 'you get what you receive' is absolutely true in my opinion.

Like the Food Diary, don't go crazy on what to catalog in the Exercise Diary during the first few weeks; keep it simple, write entries, like, "I walked for 5 minutes today, and when I got home, I had a knee pain, and I was out of breath."

Simple entries. As you get fitter and more complex training is incorporated into your exercise, you can be more comprehensive and more detailed, for example, "I runaround the football field 6 times today, I average 3 minutes per lap, no injuries nor pain, felt good."

I think you get the idea.

Weight Loss Tip Number 39– Set Goals and work "Religiously" to accomplish them.

Now it's all in our head, if we sit in front of the TV all day watching movies, or watching sports, or basically watching other people doing the things we desire, dream, or want, then nothing is going to get done.

I used to be like that; I wanted to try something, but as soon as I saw someone else doing it, it would destroy the mystery for me because I would stop seeing it as a challenge anymore.

Don't be like that, as I was back then. Challenge yourself, stop watching TV, and also stop wasting time in front of the computer.

Set a Goal, break it into smaller Goals so it will not be as intimidating, and then find the time and manage your life around accomplishing those mini goals. With every small goal or sub-goal you achieve, you are getting closer to your dream or desire Goal. It is only when you climb all the steps of the ladder that you are on the top, and it will not be a dream or desire anymore but a reality!

Start educating yourself on time management, start training your mind to solve goal-oriented problems. Everything is practice, and practice does make you perfect.

Change your mindset; free yourself from the slavery of DOING NOTHING and also the prison of WISHFUL THINKING.

Get your life back, design a project and start doing it, work on it and finish it.

Weight Loss Tip Number 40– Never stop searching and questioning.

Now, somebody will ask me how on earth searching and questioning will make me lose weight. Well, it's simple; ignorance kills if you are overweight or obese like I was a few years ago. Therefore, I know what I am talking about when I tell you that you are fat because you lack the knowledge to change your way you think about food and exercise.

You are not overweight or obese because your DNA says you are; you are overweight because you don't know how to eat right, and you don't know how to feed your body with the correct nutrients.

Six years ago, I was fat and depressed – these two usually go together. It was when I started educating myself on nutrition, and fortunately on getting nutrition from a whole, unrefined, plant-based diet, and then turned it into a lifestyle, that I started seeing tangible results. The fat around my waste started to disappear.

Applying this lifestyle combined with running were and still are my two secrets of success.

I lost the pounds safely, healthy, and never gained them back, and as long as I keep this healthy lifestyle, I will never go back to be overweight, obese, and miserable.

Start by acknowledging that you don't know anything about nutrition, that you can get your protein and also your calcium from plant-based sources; you don't need meat, you don't need other animal dairy products.

Search and question everything. Come on people, we live in a capitalistic society, the companies that sell these products are only after your money; they don't care if you get sick! Wake up!!!

It's the same scenario with Tobacco smoking; it took 7000 scientific research papers and scientific research to force the General Surgeon of America to step up and say smoking does kill people.

You know why it's harder now to get the Surgeon General to come out and say meat and dairy and generally animal products are killing you from inside out? Because Tobacco companies compared to BIG MEAT, BIG COMPANIES it's a midget, economically speaking.

We are talking about a LOT of MONEY here!!!

Also, the pharmaceutical companies will lose a huge load of money if people started eating a more plant-based diet; most of the so-called chronic diseases out there and a lot of types of cancers, like colorectal cancer today, are a direct result of animal product consumption, especially processed meat consumption.

Imagine a world without high blood pressure, with no high cholesterol, no heart attacks, no need for bypass surgery and so on.

The answer to why we are still not properly informed that animal products are not good for us is plain and simple: greed and money, power and money, control and money.

Weight Loss Tip Number 41– Be a little selfish.

If you want to change the way you look, if you want to change the way you feel, as I covered in this article, you need first to change your mindset, you need to change the way you think about certain aspects of your life.

First, you need to educate yourself about nutrition, especially about whole plant-based nutrition.

Second, you need to start applying lifestyle changes as exercise is concerned; stop the love-hate relationship you have with your TV or your computer and commit yourself to start adopting a training program that will keep you fit and healthy in the long run.

In order to even start considering all the things I just mentioned, you need to be a little bit selfish. You need to stop feeling guilty that if you do something for yourself, you will let down your husband, spouse, boyfriend or girlfriend. You need to stop feeling guilty that you might disappoint your kids by taking some time for yourself and not spending that time with them.

Let me ask you something. Your husband, spouse, boyfriend and your kids or pets, your wife, your girlfriend and your parents, what do you think they want, a person that is healthy and happy or someone that at any moment is at risk of having a stroke or a heart attack or that they are depressed or miserable? No, they want a person that is healthy, so they can do activities together, and they want you to be around for many years to come.

So, let that selfish gene kick in; program, plan, and apply a nutritional and exercise regime that will enable you to change your life for the better.

Weight Loss Tip Number 42– A journey starts with a small step.

This sentence, "a journey starts with a small step" is so absolutely true for me, and I saw it firsthand that it is indeed the case.

The reason that I wrote this article is that I really want to help people understand that first you need to change your way of thinking, that's why many of my tips here have to do with that.

If you manage to do that, then the world is yours.

I speak from the heart, I speak the truth, I am honest with you. I have nothing to gain from you, well, except of course if you want to buy my books, that would be nice, but other than that, I am not selling you a diet program or an exercise machine that would miraculously make you think and give you a six pack in a month!

The reason that I give 42 tips is that this year, September 8, I will turn 42 years old, and I have to tell you, folks, I couldn't be feeling better as health and happiness are concerned. Well, apart from the sadness I'm feeling these days because I'm going through a post-divorce period, my health was never better.

Ten years ago, I was a chain smoker, a couch potato and I was diagnosed with stomach and duodenum ulcer, chronic constipation, heartburns, hemorrhoids and, generally speaking, I was a mess, I was 31, and I was feeling 50!

Now, I am 42, and I feel like 25!

Seven years ago, I was overweight and flirting with obesity, my cholesterol and triglycerides levels were off the chart, and I was a strong candidate for heart failure, stroke, diabetes 2, and many others so-called meat-consumption-based chronic illnesses.

I am telling you all these to show you that it does take only a small step to start a beautiful journey that will literally save your life– and the step I am referring to doesn't necessarily mean a literally physical one.

It could be the fact that you are reading these lines to be the first step in your mind towards your health saga. The fact that you are here reading an article about how to lose weight indicates that you already took the first step, and you are at the start of your journey towards a more healthy and happy human being. I salute you for your decision, and I wish you all the best.

Have a healthy and happy day!

My warmest regards,

Andreas Michaelides

Other books by Andreas Michaelides

My weight loss journey: How I lost 44 pounds and never gained them back using a plant based diet

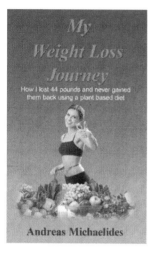

Although I never expected to drag myself out of the house and go for a run, after I finished those first three rounds at the high school track in my village, everything changed. I was so exhausted—which was an indicator of how lacking my physical fitness was—but after all the discomfort, itching, and rash in various places due to friction from excess fat, for the first time, I felt renewed, and memories of running and coming in first place in high school reminded me of how I used to be compared to how I was after those three laps around the track.

It made my eyes water; I was alone in the middle of the track under an April sky full of stars when tears of mixed feelings started pouring down from my eyes. Emotionally and psychologically, it was a turning point for me, and it also made me even more determined to become that lean, mean running machine I used to be. It was right there in that single moment that I saw the path I had to follow.

Please write a review.

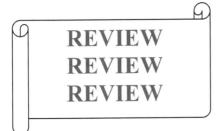

I consider myself as a person that wants to think that I am constantly improving my books, my work and myself. I am always trying to deliver to my readers the best quality and current information out there as my area of interest and expertise is concern which is Health, Nutrition and Exercise.

In order to accomplish that I need feedback from you and the only feedback I know that will help me achieve a relative perfection in all areas of my life is your valuable reviews so I know where I am wrong or where I have made mistakes and errors.

There is no such thing as a perfect book out there, perfection for one person is a sloppy work for other, so in order to satisfy as much as people out there my books need to be updated regularly and it doesn't matter if it is in electronic form (kindle) or paperback form.

If you found this book useful, please leave your review with all your thoughts, don't hold back, it will only take a few minutes of your time.

If you didn't like this book, please let me know by contacting me and I will give my best shot to fix the issue.

Thank you very much,

My warmest regards

Andreas Michaelides

Printed in Great Britain
by Amazon

68797392R00038